Homemade Cleaners

30 Natural Recipes for Around the House

TABLE OF CONTENTS

Introduction

I would first like to thank and congratulate you on downloading *"Homemade Cleaners."* I can assure you that you are going to feel so much better when you replace your expensive chemical-filled commercial cleaners with natural homemade ones. You will not have to worry about causing damage to your health or environment when using your natural cleaning solutions. You will feel confident because you will know exactly what the ingredients are that you used in your homemade cleaners.

Making your own homemade cleaning products will give you a sense of comfort in knowing that unlike many commercial cleaning products they will not be filled with harmful chemicals and toxins. Choosing to make your own natural cleaning products will make your home environment a much healthier and safer place to be—there is nothing like coming home to a clean and healthy home environment. To help you to make these positive changes you will find some easy-to-follow recipes for all kinds of home cleaning products within these pages.

Chapter 1. Mainstream Cleaning Products Are Affecting Our Health

The last thing that any of us what to imagine is that the products that we are using to keep our home environment clean could be causing more harm than good. The harmful effects of mainstream cleaning products have only recently been explored and researched in an in-depth level. Our generation has seen major increases in the prevalence of thyroid disease, cancer, asthma and infertility. Researchers are connecting the dots regarding these diseases with our enormous exposure to harmful chemicals. In the world of today we are exposed to pesticides, toxic metals, artificial food, environmental pollution, and toxic plastics just to name a few. The extreme level of the use of harmful chemicals being used daily is the reason that researching the effect on the human body has been very challenging to conduct.

When it comes to mainstream cleaning products ingredients most of the them have been identified as major culprits in affecting our health. We are exposed to these chemicals slowly over a long period, our generation has experienced the results of this first hand.

Looking back in human history to the Queen Victoria Era is a strange but visible example of what chemicals can do to the body over long periods of time. During this era, the nobles used to eat and drink out of silver plates and cups, in time, due to the colloidal silver ingested on a large scale, these nobles' blood acquired a blue tint—hence the term 'blue bloods' when referring to royalty.

The harmful chemicals that can be found in many of today's cleaning products on the market can be divided into three categories, namely **neurotoxins, carcinogens, and endocrine disruptors**

1. ***Neurotoxins*** are very destructive substances that cause damage to our nerve tissue, which can potentially have negative affects on our memory, concentration abilities, and sleeping patterns.
2. ***Carcinogens*** are dangerous cancer causing substances, directly affecting our bodies at a cellular level.

3. ***Endocrine Disruptors*** interfere with our hormone systems, this in turn causes our bodies to respond erratically to these mixed signals.

You may feel a bit betrayed by those cleaning brands that you have been using for years. Most of us have been lulled into believing that the mainstream cleaning products we are using are completely safe. We feel that the authorities certainly would not allow cleaning product companies to produce harmful products that could very well be responsible for causing diseases. The sad truth is that many companies are driven by profit, for many they would have to shut their doors without the use of these chemicals. The authorities are not able to intervene unless there is rock solid proof that a specific substance, is a potential health risk.

Not only are many mainstream cleaning products harmful to our health but they are also extremely detrimental to the environment. Most mainstream aerosol spray cans contain CFC's that cause harm to the ozone layer and contribute to the greenhouse effect. Our future is pointing to us heading towards a global water crisis, adding to this crisis is toxic substances from cleaning products finding their way into sensitive water systems, causing harm to our natural resources on a large scale long after you wash them down your kitchen sink.

You must act against mainstream cleaning products to help provide a healthier environment and help in ensuring the long-term wellbeing of yourself and loved ones.

Good News:

It is not difficult to go green. You will certainly be able to enjoy the health benefits and peace of mind, along with the fact that all-natural cleaning products are very cost effective that you can totally customize to your personal needs. The green recipes within these pages are 100% safe to use around young children and pets, their eco friendly ingredients do not harm the body or environment in any way.

Chapter 2. Covering the Basics of Natural Cleaners

Here is your introduction into the wonderful world of natural cleaning products. The ingredients have quite the job as they need to be safe for the human body, biodegradable, cost effective and work just as well or better than their chemical opponents.

The following ingredients you will find in most of the cleaning solution recipes in this book:

- Olive oil
- Fresh lemons
- White vinegar
- Baking soda
- Borax
- Essential oils
- Washing soda
- Castile soap

Olive Oil

Olive oil is obtained from pressing whole olives, the oil is used in beauty products, cooking and pharmaceutical products for many years. Olive oil works great at helping to maintain leather and wooden furniture.

Fresh Lemons

Lemons are a great cleaner with amazing disinfectant abilities with the bonus of the fresh, citrus odor. Lemon juice contains high levels of citric acid, alkaline, and antibacterial agent.

White Vinegar

Vinegar is used as a condiment all over the world. It is also one of the most versatile natural cleaners you can get. White vinegar, or distilled vinegar, is basically a weak form of acetic acid, formed by a fermentation process. It has many different uses.

Borax

There has been some controversy surrounding this ingredient in natural cleaning products, due largely to the fact that many people are not very familiar with borax, commonly confusing it with boric acid. Borax is a mineral of boron, it is also referred to as sodium tetraborate, which is mined from naturally occurring seasonal lakes in Turkey, United States, and Chile amongst others. Borax is a very effective and natural substitute for chemical detergents, it will not cause cancer or other harmful conditions, it cannot be absorbed through the skin, it is perfectly fine to use in your house for a natural cleaning product.

Baking Soda

Natron is a naturally occurring substance that baking soda can be found in, consisting mainly of sodium carbonate. The ancient Egyptians used it for decades, and even used to create paint for their hieroglyphics. Today it is commercially mined in Colorado, it offers a massive range of applications, especially in cleaning solutions due to its great ability to neutralize odors and cut through grease.

Essential Oils

Essential oils are very essential in offering us a wide range of benefits. They offer strong antibacterial, antifungal, and antiviral properties, along with an array of health benefits and natural cures for many ailments. The essential oils commonly used in cleaners are

lavender, lemon, tea tree, eucalyptus, and peppermint. Most recipes only require a few
drops of essential oils, as they are very concentrated and strong.

Washing Soda

Washing soda is also referred to as sodium carbonate, it is closely related to baking
soda. It is a sodium salt of carbonic acid. It is extracted from the ashes of plants
growing in sodium soils found in the Middle East, or in the seaweed of Spain and
Scotland. One of the most important uses for it is in the manufacturing of glass. For
cleaning uses it is a useful general detergent that works great as a laundry booster.

Castile Soap

Castile is a vegetable based soap, it is traditionally made from olive oil and named after
the Castile region of Spain where it originated. Castile soap will effectively fight grime
and grease, it is used in many recipes in its liquid form.

Chapter 3. Natural Kitchen Cleaning Solutions

Kitchen

I have found that the kitchen is often the most stubborn room in the house to keep clean. Kitchens are the heart of activity in most households, with cooking, drinking, eating, interactions between family members going on, contributing to the build-up of grease and grime. The kitchen is a great area of your home to use natural cleaning products. Consider that everything that you and your loved ones consume comes into contact with the kitchen surfaces and utensils, which will inevitably be exposed to the cleaners that you use to clean them. This is a great reason for you to choose to use 100% natural and harmless products to clean your home environment—it will give you peace of mind.

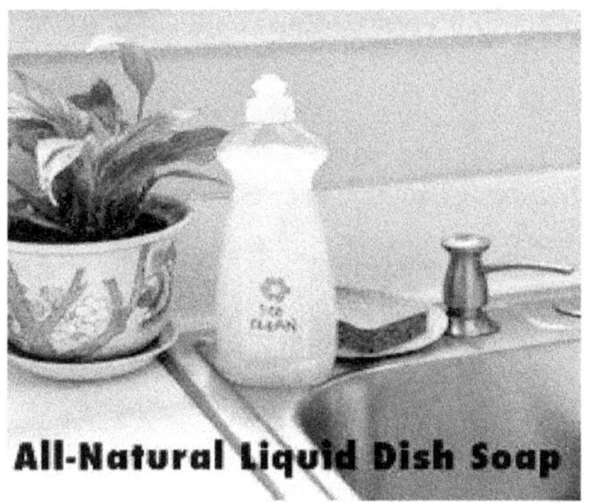

1. *Natural Dishwashing Liquid*
   Preparation time: 15-20 minutes

   Container: Glass or plastic container

   Ingredients:

   - 40 drops of essential oil of your choice (lemon, orange, or lavender work well)
   - 1 teaspoon of vegetable glycerine
   - 2 teaspoons washing soda
   - 60ml Castile soap, grated
   - 60ml Castile soap, liquid
   - 500ml boiling water

Directions:

Using a large pot, bring the water to a boil. Add in the grated Castile soap and stir it until it has dissolved. Add in the glycerine, liquid Castile soap, washing soda and stir well. Remove from heat and slowly add in the essential oils and stir to blend. Add to suitable container and allow to cool for a few hours before using.

Uses

You will find that this natural dishwashing liquid will have your dishes clean and grime free, without leaving a residue and it gentle on your hands too!

Note

Your results could vary due to the varying water hardness in different areas. If you find that the liquid is to thick simply add a bit of water to it. If you find it to be too thin, add it back into the pot on the stove and add in more washing soda. Write down your adjustments for future use.

2. Dishwasher Detergent

Preparation time: 5 minutes

Container: glass or plastic container

Ingredients:

- 2 teaspoons fresh lemon juice
- 250ml water
- 250ml Castile soap, liquid
- White vinegar

Directions:

In a container mix your fresh lemon juice, Castile soap, and water. Add this mixture to the one half of your dishwasher's detergent compartment, and fill the other half with white vinegar.

Uses

The combination of the fresh lemon juice and the Castile soap will degrease and kill germs, while the vinegar rinse will leave them sparkling.

Notes

You should always check the built-in salt level of your dishwasher. This is essential in working to prevent streaks on glasses and leaving a nice grease free finish.

3. Natural Pot & Pan Cleaner

Preparation time: 5 to 10 minutes

Container: No need for container apply ingredients directly to your dirty pots and pans.

Ingredients:

- 2 tablespoons baking soda
- 250ml white vinegar
- Coarse sea salt
- Hot water
- Stiff brush or pot scourer

Directions:

This is a two-step process, depending on how dirty the pot or pan is, this method will also work with burnt pan. For mild grease, you can sprinkle some coarse sea salt all over the surface, add hot water and clean with stiff brush. If this does not work, then place the pot or pan on stove and fill with hot water. Add in about 250ml of white vinegar. Bring this mix to a boil. Remove from the stove and add 2 tablespoons of baking soda. Watch the grease fizz away before your eyes! Rinse, if you still have some grease, add neat baking soda and clean with hot water and a stiff brush.

Uses

You can use this method for any pot or pan, even those that have baked on food and stubborn grease, or even a burnt pan.

4. Fridge & Freezer Cleaner

Preparation time: 5 minutes

Container: bucket of hot water is all you will need

Ingredients:

- 125ml baking soda
- 1 bucket hot water
- Fresh lemon juice

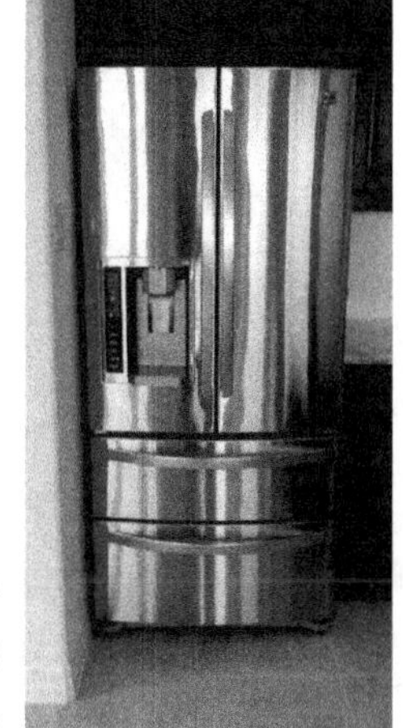

Directions:

This is often a very dirty exercise, since most of us do not clean out our fridges very often. Baking soda is a great help in this chore. Just dip a cloth in your mixture and apply it to all the nooks and crevices you need to clean inside of your fridge. For a fresh touch go over the inside of your fridge with some fresh lemon juice and wipe it clean with a cloth. The lemon juice will help kill germs and leave your fridge smelling fresh and clean.

Uses

This method can be used on any king of fridge or freezer.

Notes

If your fridge has an ice or water dispenser built into it, you can use a clean cloth dipped in vinegar to wipe down the inside. Wipe with a damp cloth afterwards, and run some water through to prevent your drinks from tasting like vinegar.

5. Oven & Stove Cleaner

Preparation time:* 15 *minutes

Container: Apply directly to stubborn grime on your stove or oven.

Ingredients:

- Baking soda
- Vinegar

Directions:

Heat your oven to 130⁰ C and spray neat vinegar generously on areas with stubborn grease and grime. Take the baking soda and sprinkle it over the same areas and leave it on for a few minutes. Turn off your oven and allow it to cool. Use a wet sponge or cloth to wipe away the mess. Use this same method for the stove, just without heat.

Uses

This recipe can also be applied to outdoor grills or just about anything that needs some intense removal of dirt and grime. Even when you do not heat up this solution it will still degrease.

6. Counter Top Cleaner I

Preparation time: 5 minutes

Container: glass or plastic spray bottle

Ingredients:

- Water
- Baking soda

Directions:

In a spray bottle add four tablespoons of baking soda with one litre of warm water.

Uses

Baking soda works well on dissolving dirt without much effort on your part. Spray this mix on your counter tops and wipe them with a cloth or sponge.

Notes

This is a safe recipe to use on all surfaces, including granite, stone and marble.

7. Counter Top Cleaner II
Preparation time: 5 minutes

Container: glass or plastic spray bottle

Ingredients:

- Water
- White vinegar

Directions:

Mix the ingredients in equal parts in a spray bottle.

Uses

This easy to prepare spray works great for cleaning your kitchen counter tops. The vinegar will cut through the grease and grime, leaving your counter tops shining, wipe with damp cloth.

Notes

If you have stone, marble or granite countertops you can substitute the vinegar with rubbing alcohol or vodka, that will do a similar attack on the grease and grime without damaging your counter tops.

8. Mildew Remover

Preparation time: 5 minutes

Container: Add mixture to spray bottle

Ingredients:

- Tea tree essential oil
- Vinegar
- Fresh lemon juice

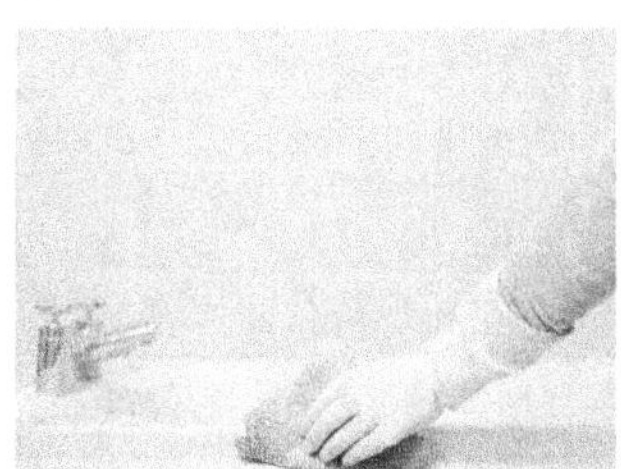

Directions:

The most common area in a kitchen to find mildew is under a leaky basin or anywhere that gets moisture and not much sun. The two main ingredients in your natural mildew remover of tea tree essential oil and vinegar will get rid of the mildew in no time. First you need to apply the vinegar using a spray bottle, undiluted. After a few hours if there are still some stubborn mould patches, make a mix of 500ml of water and 40 drops of tea tree oil in a spray bottle, a. Shake the bottle well before using and apply to mouldy area.

Uses

You can store your unused tea tree mixture indefinitely. It is a great broad spectrum mould killer. It also works well on shower curtains, mouldy ceilings, or even musty carpets and rugs.

Notes

In the bathroom recipe section, there is an alternative mould removal recipe. Use whatever one works best for you.

9. Cutting Boards Cleaner

Preparation time: 5 minutes

Container: no container is needed

Ingredients:

- 1 fresh lemon
- Coarse sea salt

Directions:

This is a wonderful and simple recipe to help sanitize your kitchen cutting board. Cut a fresh lemon in half, sprinkle coarse salt all over the cutting board and run the lemon over the salt. Squish the lemon to get out as much lemon juice as you can, allow it to sit for about 10 minutes. Rinse cutting board with warm water. Job done!

Uses

You can apply this method to any cutting or chopping board, wooden or plastic.

10. Unclogging the Kitchen Sink
Preparation time: **10-15 minutes**

Container: Pour directly into the sink

Ingredients:

- 250ml white vinegar
- 500ml boiling water
- 500ml baking soda

Directions:

Begin the process by pouring 250ml of baking soda down the clogged drain. Follow with the boiling water. Give it a few minutes to do its job. Add another 250ml of baking soda followed with 250ml of white vinegar and quickly plug the drain. You will hear the gunk fizzing away inside the drain. After a few minutes, flush with some more boiling water.

Uses

You can use this method to unclog your drain or use it to prevent your drain from becoming clogged by applying it regularly.

Notes

If you find that your drain is still clogged after using this method, you might want to consider using a plunger. This method may have loosened the sludge but the plunger can help to encourage it to come out.

11. Microwave Cleaner

Preparation time: 5 minutes

Container: any microwaveable bowl is fine

Ingredients:

- Lemon juice
- Vinegar

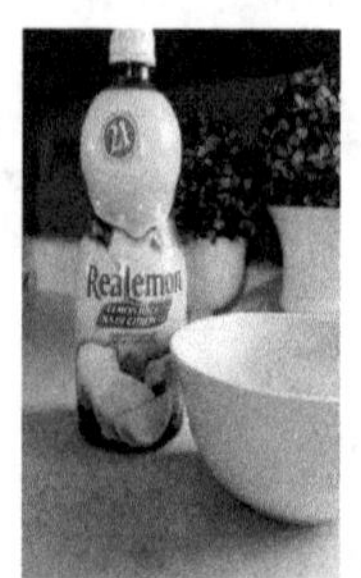

Directions:

This is a fast and easy way to clean your microwave. Fill the bowl with vinegar and mix in a few drops of lemon juice. Microwave mix on high for 2 minutes, leave microwave sealed up for a few minutes before you open the door. Using a cloth to wipe down the inside of your microwave it will look great in no time and will be germ free!

12. *Essential Oil Air Freshener*
Preparation time: 5 minutes

Container: You will need a tea light candle and an essential oil burner.

Ingredients:

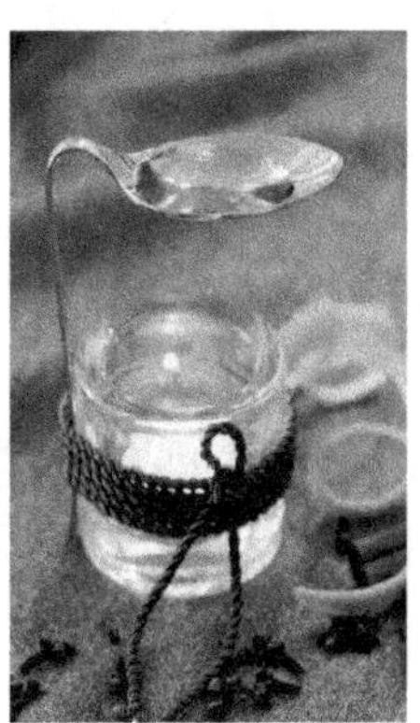

- Essential oils
- Water

Directions:

Add a bit of water to your oil tray of your burner, light the tea light candle underneath. To freshen the air, add the following blend of essential oils to the water:

- Five drops of lemon essential oil
- 10 drops of lavender essential oil
- 3 drops of lime essential oil
- 3 drops of grapefruit essential oil

Make sure to put out the tea light as soon as the burner dries up and the oil has been vaporized.

Uses

This is a wonderful way that you can add a lasting fragrance into your home, especially after cleaning to freshen the air.

Notes

You can also use essential oil diffusers for the same purpose.

13. Natural Laminate Floor Cleaner

Preparation time: 5 minutes

Container: pour ingredients into cleaning bucket

Ingredients:

- White vinegar
- Hot water
- Essential oil

Directions:

Fill your cleaning bucket with half hot water and half white vinegar, and mix well. Add in a few drops of eucalyptus or peppermint essential oils, and the mixture is ready to clean your laminate floor.

14. Furniture Polish

Preparation time: 5-10 minutes

Container: any suitable container

Ingredients:

- 180ml olive oil
- 60ml white vinegar

Directions:

Blend the ingredients in a container and apply sparingly to your furniture using a soft cloth, until the desired effect is achieved.

Uses

This mix can be used to freshen up all your furniture around the house.

Notes

You can replace the white vinegar with 60ml of lemon juice following the same method as above.

15. Wall Scrub

Preparation time: 5 minutes

Container: any suitable plastic container or glass

Ingredients:

- White vinegar
- Warm water

Directions:

Blend the 60ml of vinegar in a cleaning bucket along with warm water.

Uses

Use this mix to clean walls and get rid of scuff marks using a cloth or sponge.

Notes

For those stubborn marks on your walls, add some baking soda and scrub the problem area.

16. Carpet Stain Remover I
Preparation time: 3 months

Container: large glass bottle or jar

Ingredients:

- Fresh peels of orange and lemon
- Brown sugar
- Water

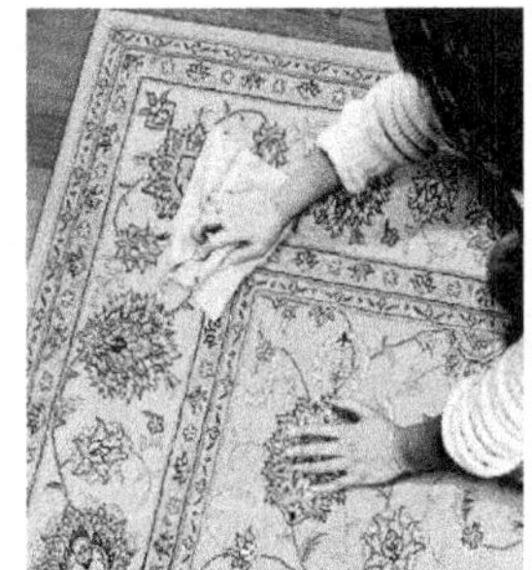

Directions:

This recipe will help you to create your own powerful stain remover, it relies on enzymes to biologically digest and eat away odours and stains. Pour 100ml of brown sugar into your glass container, add in 375ml of fresh citrus peels, fill with water and tightly seal the container and give it a good shake. Release the cap about halfway to release gases during the process. Wait for 3 months.

Uses

Works great on stubborn stains, just pour this enzymatic cleaner onto stain and wipe up with cloth 20 minutes later.

17. Carpet Stain Remover II
Preparation time: *5 minutes*

Container: *glass or plastic spray bottle*

Ingredients:

- 60ml baking
- 500ml white vinegar
- 500ml warm water

Directions:

Before applying the stain remover, try to get as much of the staining substance off the carpet as possible. Use some kitchen towels or wet cloth or sponge. In a large bowl, mix warm water and vinegar, followed by the baking soda. Pour this mix into spray bottle and thoroughly wet the strained area. Leave it to soak for 10 minutes, then rub off with damp cloth.

Uses

This stain remover will work on things such blood stains, and urine, it will also remove odors.

18. Carpet Cleaning Powder
Preparation time: 5 minutes

Container: glass jar

Ingredients:

- 18 drops essential oils
- 250ml baking soda
- 125 ml borax

Directions:

In a glass jar, mix baking soda and borax thoroughly and drip in 6 drops of lavender, peppermint, tea tree essential oils. This mixture disinfects, repels bugs and has a nice fresh clean smell. Shake contents to mix oils into powder.

Uses

Sprinkle powder over any carpet that needs a little freshening up. Let it sit for about 20 minutes before you vacuum it up.

19. Simple Tile Cleaner

Preparation time: 5 minutes

Container: mix in cleaning bucket

Ingredients:

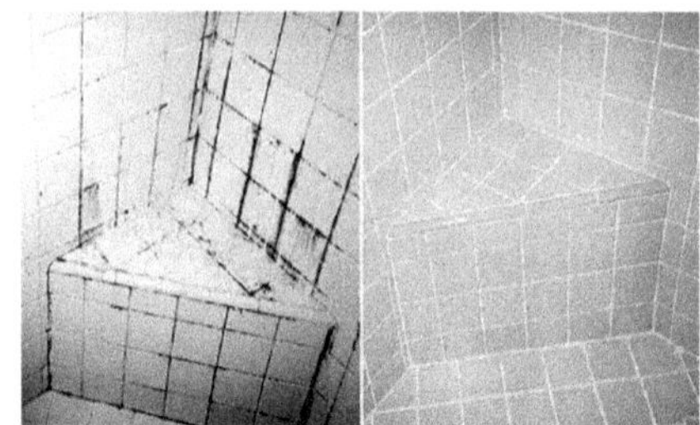

- White vinegar
- Lemon essential oil
- Warm water

Directions:

Fill one third of bucket with white vinegar and top it off with warm water. Add 20 drops of lemon essential oil. Wash the floors with this solution using a rag or mop-best part is that you do not need to rinse it off. It is going to leave your floors looking shiny and free from dirt and grime.

Uses

This recipe is perfect for regular cleaning of tiles throughout the house.

Notes

I would recommend this method for any kind of wooden floors.

Chapter 5. Homemade Laundry Cleaning Products

20. Fabric Softener
Preparation time: 5 minutes

Container: any suitable glass jar

Ingredients:

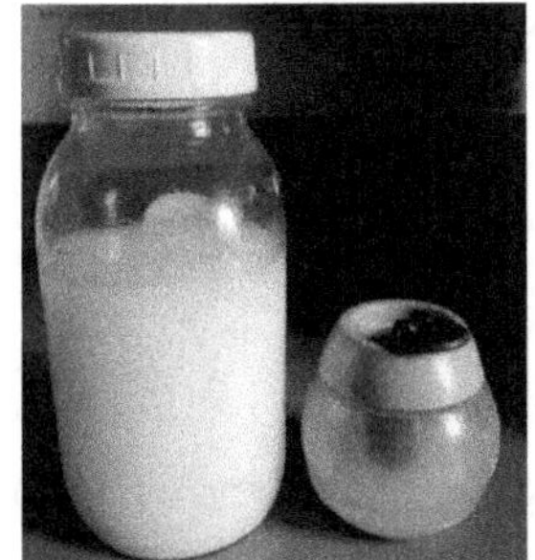

- 10 drops of essential oil
- 1 litre of white vinegar

Directions:

In a glass container pour in 10 drops of essential oil and one litre of white vinegar. Using lavender or lemon essential oils works well when it comes to laundry. Shake well before each use.

Use

Add between 125 to 250ml to a rinse cycle, depending on the load size.

21. Keeping Moths Away

Preparation time: 5 minutes

Ingredients:

- ***Fresh lemon peels***

Directions:

This wonderful tip will prevent moths from moving into your closet and nibbling on your clothes. Simply add some fresh lemon peel to your cupboards and replace them every couple of weeks.

22. Natural Laundry Detergent—Liquid

Preparation time: 20 minutes

Container: suitable glass jars

Ingredients:

- 250ml borax
- 250ml washing soda
- 250ml liquid Castile soap
- 15 drops of essential oil

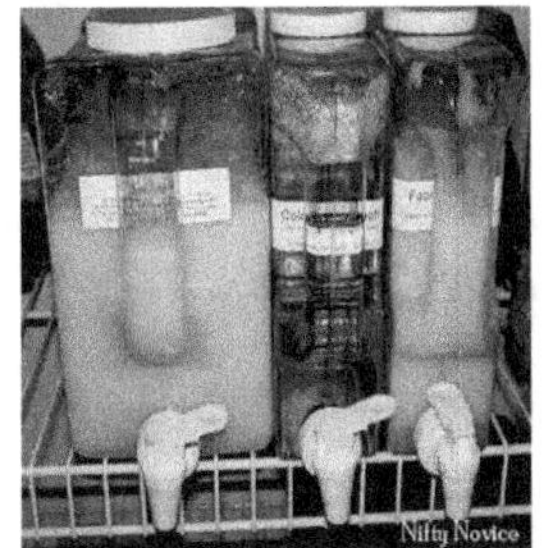

Directions:

In a large pot boil one and a half litres of water. As the water starts to boil, turn off the heat and add borax and washing soda. Stir thoroughly. In a bucket, mix the liquid Castile soap with two and a half litres of room temperature water. Add the essential oil of your choice to add a nice aroma to your detergent. Pour the heated mixture from the stove to the bucket and stir. Now, pour your natural liquid laundry detergent into the suitable glass jars to store it in.

Uses

Use about 60ml of liquid detergent per laundry load.

Notes

For removal of stains, you can use some liquid detergent directly on the stain and let it sit for awhile before washing with the rest of your load.

23. Natural Laundry Detergent Powder
Preparation time: 5-10 minutes

Container: large glass jar

Ingredients:

- Washing soda
- Castile soap bar
- Baking soda
- Borax

Directions:

Grate your Castile soap bar into fine flakes. In your jar add 400ml washing soda, 400ml of borax, and 200ml grated Castile soap. Sprinkle a few teaspoons of baking soda over the mixture. Close the jar and shake to mix your ingredients.

Uses

Use 60ml of your laundry detergent mix per laundry load.

24. Cockroaches

Preparation time: 5 minutes

Container: small glass bowl or container

Ingredients:

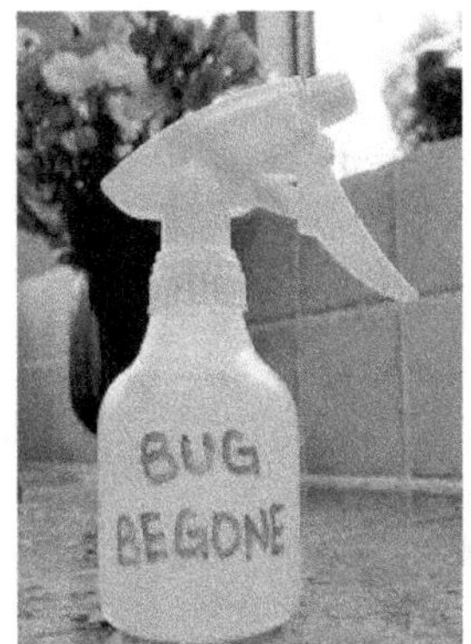

- Baking soda
- Borax
- Epsom salts

Directions:

Mix together 100ml of baking soda, borax, and Epsom salts. Leave the unsealed container on the counters or in cabinets to repel cockroaches.

25. Bedbugs

Preparation time: 10-30 minutes

Container: any suitable spray bottle

Ingredients:

- Fresh garlic
- Tea tree essential oil
- Rosemary essential oil
- Rose geranium essential oil
- Distilled water

Directions:

First give your linen a 20-minute cycle in the dryer if you are having problems with bedbugs. In a spray bottle, fill with water and drip into it 5 drops of tea tree oil, add a few cloves of fresh garlic, 5 drops of rosemary essential oil, 5 drops of rose geranium essential oil. Shake well before each use apply a fine mist on the mattress and bedding, allow it to dry out. Repeat the process at least three consecutive days.

26. Ticks & Fleas-Pets
Preparation time: 5-10 minutes

Container: any spray bottle

Ingredients:

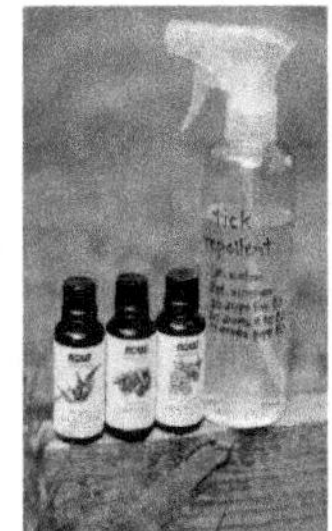

- lavender, tea tree, and rose geranium essential oils
- distilled water
- white vinegar

Directions:

Fill your spray bottle about halfway with distilled water, top off with vinegar. Drip in 5 drops of lavender, 5 drops of tea tree, 5 drops of rose geranium essential oils and shake before using.

Uses

You can use this to repel insects by lightly spraying it onto your pet's fur. Repeat if problem persists.

Notes

Test a small are of your pet's skin to make sure its skin is not sensitive to it.

27. Mosquito and Flies

Preparation time: 5-10 minutes

Container: any suitable spray bottle

Ingredients:

- Sweet almond oil
- Vodka
- Lemon essential oil
- Eucalyptus essential oil
- Lavender essential oil
- Rosemary essential oil

Directions:

Add 30ml of vodka to a spray bottle along with 30ml of sweet almond oil. Drip in 50 drops of lemon eucalyptus essential oil, 15 drops of rosemary essential oil, 15 drops of lavender essential oil, and mix well. Shake before you spray.

Uses

Spray in a room or directly on your skin for protection from flying insects.

28. Ants—Natural Repelling Methods
Preparation time: 5-10 minutes

Ingredients:

- Fresh cucumber
- Cayenne pepper
- Dried mint leaves
- Cloves

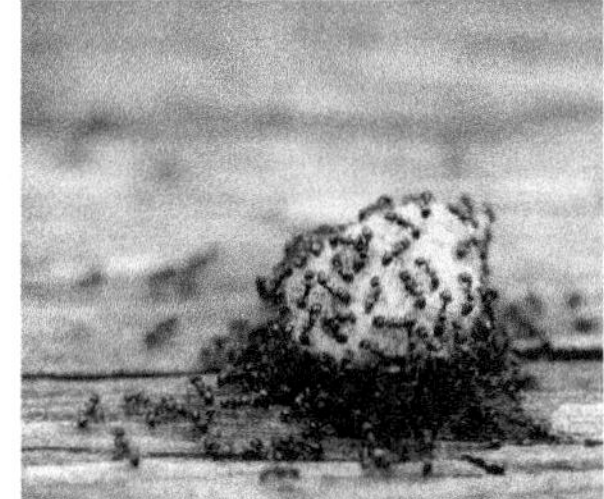

Directions:

Try a combination of these methods to stop them from entering your home. Sprinkle cayenne pepper across entry points into your home, especially add to spots where you see a line of ants entering your home. Leave dried mint leaves, cloves and slices of fresh cucumber at the edges of counters this will help discourage the ants from exploring further.

29. General Insect Repellent
Preparation time: 14 days

Container: Sealable 1 litre glass jar or container

Ingredients:

- 1 litre of apple cider vinegar
- Dried herbs: mint, thyme, rosemary, lavender, and sage

Directions:

Add into glass container two tablespoons of dried herbs and apple cider vinegar. Seal the container and shake the mixture daily for 14 consecutive days. Strain to remove the herbs and pour it into a spray bottle for easy application.

Uses

Store this mix in the fridge and use it when you experience a bug infestation in your home.

Notes

To use the mix on your skin dilute it with equal parts of water.

30. Alternative General Insect Repellant
Preparation time: 5 minutes

Container: Any suitable spray bottle

Ingredients:

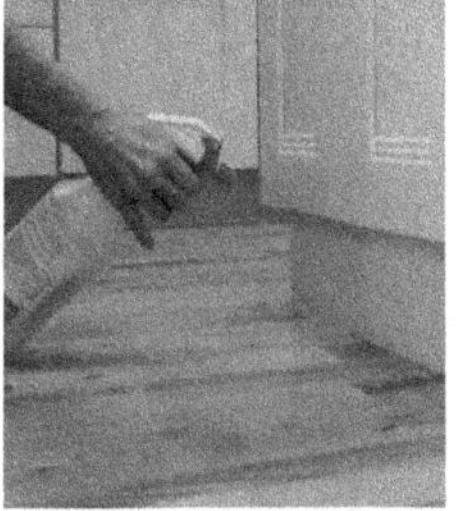

- Distilled water
- Essential oils: rosemary, clove, eucalyptus, lavender and cinnamon
- Witch hazel tincture

Directions:

Fill a spray bottle halfway with water, top it up with witch hazel tincture. Add in 10 drops of each of the essential oils.

Uses

Use when you have uninvited creepy crawlies in your home.

Conclusion

I hope that this collection of natural cleaning recipes will suit your cleaning needs. You can certainly put your mind at rest in knowing that they are not filled with harmful chemicals that could be a health risk and concern to you and your loved ones. These products are not only safe and easy to prepare, but they are also very cost effective. Currently many of us are trying to live on a budget which can be very challenging. These natural cleaning recipes will help to reduce your costs in cleaning supplies significantly while be a much healthier option for you and the environment. I wish you great results in switching to using natural 'green' cleaning products—this is a positive step towards leading a healthier lifestyle!

I Need Your Support...

Thanks again for reading my book and supporting my work, I truly hope that you gained great value from its contents. If you indeed did find value in this book, then I would like to ask a favor of you, I would really be grateful to you if you would leave a review of this book on Amazon.

FREE BONUS REMINDER

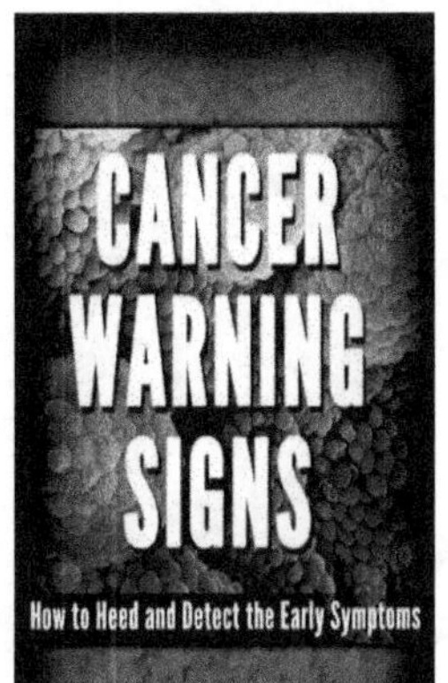

If you have not grabbed it yet, please go ahead and download your special bonus report *"Cancer Warning Signs. How To Heed & Detect The Early Symptoms!"*
Simply Click the Button Below

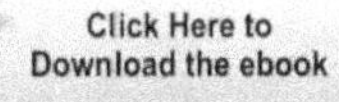

OR **Go to This Page**
http://healthylivingpeople.com/free/

BONUS #2: More Free & Discounted Books or Products
Do you want to receive more Free/Discounted Books or Products?

We have a mailing list where we send out our new Books or Products when they go free or with a discount on Amazon. Click on the link below to sign up for Free & Discount Book & Product Promotions.
=> Sign Up for Free & Discount Book & Product Promotions <=

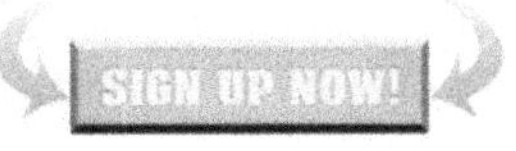

OR Go to this URL
http://zbit.ly/1WBb1Ek